Injury Prevention Movement

Volume 1

Core Concepts and Posture

LINCOLN BLANDFORD

Performance Matrix Team

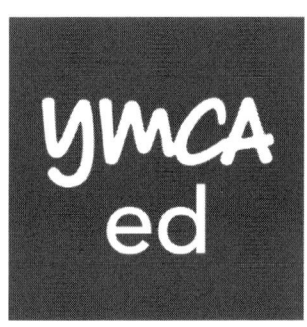

Discover more books and ebooks of interest to you and find out about the range of work we do at the forefront of health, fitness and wellbeing.

www.centralymcaguides.com

Injury Prevention and Movement Control Vol.1

Published by Central YMCA Trading Ltd (trading as YMCAed).
Registered Company No. 3667206.

Central YMCA is the world's founding YMCA. Established in 1844 in Central London, it was the first YMCA to open its doors and, in so doing, launched a movement that has now grown to become the world's biggest youth organisation. Today, Central YMCA is the UK's leading health, fitness and wellbeing charity, committed to helping people from all walks of life – and particularly the young and those with a specific need – to live happier, healthier and more fulfilled lives.

Copyright © Central YMCA Trading Ltd 2014
All rights reserved.

ISBN: 1495351726
ISBN-13: 978-1495351723

Central YMCA Health and Fitness Guides

DISCLAIMER

This book is presented solely for educational and entertainment purposes. The author and publisher are not offering it as legal, medical, or other professional services advice. While best efforts have been used in preparing this book, the author and publisher make no representations or warranties of any kind and assume no liabilities of any kind with respect to the accuracy or completeness of the contents and specifically disclaim any implied warranties of merchantability or fitness of use for a particular purpose. Neither the publisher nor the individual author(s) shall be liable for any physical, psychological, emotional, financial, or commercial damages, including, but not limited to, special, incidental, consequential or other damages, resulting from the information or programs contained herein. Every person is different and the information, advice and programs contained herein may not be suitable for your situation. Exercise is not without its risks and, as such, we would strongly advise that you consult with your healthcare professional before beginning any programme of exercise, especially if you have, or suspect you may have, any injuries or illnesses, are currently pregnant or have recently given birth. The advice, information and guidance given in Central YMCA Guides is in no way intended as a substitute for medical consultation. As with any form of exercise, you should stop immediately if you feel faint, dizzy or have physical discomfort or pain or any other contra-indication, and consult a physician.

This book is based on the concepts of The Performance Matrix, from Movement Performance Solutions and developed from the work of Mark Comerford and Sarah Mottram. Lincoln Blandford has interpreted these processes for a readership of fitness professionals and those interested in remaining active and injury free.

We are grateful for the contributions of Sarah Mottram, Mark Comerford, Warrick McNeill, Jeanette Hoftijzer, Clare Pedersen, Michael Nicol and Jacqueline Swart, for their input on practical application, their wealth of experience and their painstaking editing.

CONTENTS

About The Author

Inspirations and Contributions   1

Introduction   5

1   Looking For The Core?   9

2   Movement Control: The Challenges   15

3   Posture and Alignment   27

Final Summary   37

References   39

The Central YMCA Guides Series   47

ABOUT THE AUTHOR

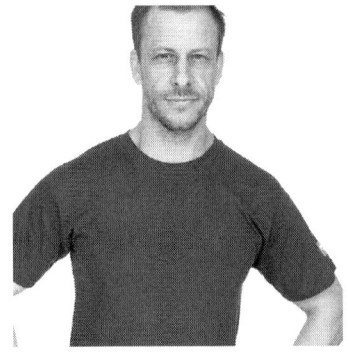

Over the past decade I have tutored over a thousand students to become successful personal trainers within the UK fitness industry. Some have remained in the UK, successfully pursuing this career, others have travelled the world. All have hopefully taken the message of the importance of movement quality and applied it to improving their clients' health and fitness, worldwide. This book aims to support both them and their clients in this worthy cause.

In addition to my teaching roles for both YMCAfit and Performance Matrix I regularly contribute to fitness media, writing on injury prevention and performance enhancement through the use of movement screening. I have developed numerous training courses for YMCAfit alongside collaborating with the Performance Matrix team in the development of their personal trainer specific 'Movement Screening Fundamentals' module. I maintain a select personal training client base within London as I continue to develop my own abilities and understanding through on-going study of Strength and Conditioning at St Mary's University College, Pilates, and yoga.

What unites these three apparently distinctly different approaches is the body and its movements. A greater understanding of both, through any chosen discipline, will empower trainers to make better decisions, evaluate questionable claims, and avoid the dogmas that stop us asking 'why?' and 'is there a better way?'.

I'm delighted that you've chosen to spend time with my book and really hope that you enjoy the reading of it, applying the ideas in it and answering the questions it may well raise.

Lincoln

Central YMCA Health and Fitness Guides

INSPIRATIONS AND CONTRIBUTIONS

Much of this text has been greatly inspired by the work of Mark Comerford and Sarah Mottram who have made significant contributions to the movement control concept, further developing the application of these ideas with post graduate rehab specialist qualifications, working alongside elite sports teams and contributing to ongoing research. Their movement control testing protocols identify the presence of uncontrolled movement, under a system known as The Performance Matrix. Although movement screening is not included in this text, I'd encourage all of you to have your movement control checked through a qualified source. As a further introduction to the concept see Blandford & Comerford (2013).

Also bringing their sizable experience to the text are other members of the Performance Matrix team. This globally based collective of movement specialists work with elite level movement professionals, employing Comerford and Mottram's movement screening systems. Additionally, the principal author has applied the highly contemporary concepts of 'movement IQ' in a fitness setting and it is from this perspective that the text is primarily composed.

SARAH MOTTRAM

Sarah Mottram is an educator, clinician and researcher who has principally focussed upon the influence of uncontrolled movement on the recurrence of pain and deficits in performance. Over the past 18 years she has lectured nationally and internationally on evidence-based solutions to better understand, prevent and manage musculoskeletal pain and injury related to movement impairments.

Sarah is particularly interested in the integration of differing movement therapies as a means of retraining uncontrolled movement, something evident through her certification in Pilates, GYROTONIC® and the highly contemporary discipline 'Garuda'. She incorporates these valuable tools in her clinical practice based at The Movement Works, in Chichester, UK.

MARK COMERFORD

In addition to being a director of Movement Performance Solutions, Mark is also world renowned in the field performance and clinical rehab, a reputation enhanced through his role as an educator and author. He delivers consultancy to various sporting and professional organisations which includes 3 NBA teams, West Side Dance and Physical Therapy (New York Ballet), Vermeil Sport & Fitness (USA) and Athletes' Performance (USA).

He has a special interest in the development of clinically relevant models of movement function and dysfunction, understanding the influence of pain on movement and muscle function and the enhancement of performance. He has published papers on movement and muscle function; the integration of local and global muscle training to enhance joint stability; and movement control training. He has frequently been invited to speak at numerous international conferences for movement based professionals around the world.

JEANNETTE HOFTIJZER

Jeannette after graduating as Physiotherapist at the Academy for Sports Studies in The Hague, Holland, Jeanette worked in Switzerland whilst continuing post graduate education culminating with her qualification as a manual therapist. Jeannette currently works in private practice and is aligned with the Johan Cruyff Institute and several other talent programmes of the Dutch Olympic Committee. Several professional track and field, speedskating, ice hockey, basketball, and tennis clubs currently utilise Jeanette as their specialist performance advisor.

MICHAEL NICOL

Originally training in Sports Rehabilitation, Michael completed a Masters in Sports Medicine at Nottingham University. He is now registered with both the Chartered Society of Physiotherapists (CSP) and The British Association of Sport Rehabilitators and Trainers (BASRaT) and clinically works at the St Mary's Clinic in London. He is also a Senior Lecturer in Sport Rehabilitation at St Mary's University College and holds the position of Director of Enterprise within the School of Sport Health and Applied Science. Michael has been involved with Movement Performance Solutions for over 10 years and through that time has both lectured and consulted within professional sport both in the UK and across Europe.

CLARE PEDERSEN

Clare is a chartered physiotherapist with extensive experience in sports medicine and return to sport following injury. She has worked in elite football and handball and was senior physiotherapist for Great Britain's orienteering team 2000-2006. She now works full time at Arena Fysio in Helsingborg, Sweden screening and retraining recreational and elite athletes in many sports. Clare is also a Performance Matrix Accredited Instructor, and delivers Performance Matrix courses In Sweden and throughout Europe.

WARRICK MCNEILL

Warrick is a New Zealand trained physiotherapist, currently running a physiotherapy clinic that operates out of a well-established Pilates studio in Central London. Qualified in Pilates himself, Warrick has a keen interest in treating performers, particularly dancers, which has led to his involvement with the Physiotherapy Advisory Committee to Dance UK, the Royal National Theatre and the Royal Shakespeare Company. He regularly presents to Pilates training organisations, dancers and dance teachers and possesses a keen interest in ergonomics and its use in the workplace. He has taught courses internationally for The Performance Matrix and is an associate editor of the 'Journal of Bodywork and Movement Therapies'.

JACQUELINE SWART

Jacqueline lectures on the 'Orthopaedic Manual Therapy' course within a South African university. She has delivered various rehabilitation courses for physiotherapists and presented at movement therapy based symposiums and conferences over the last 15 years. Alongside her role of treating and subsequently training athletes, Jacqueline has a special interest in injury prevention. She teaches courses for both The Performance Matrix and Kinetic Control and has been using The Performance Matrix system for assessment and successfully integrating Pilates exercise in to athletes' rehabilitation. In 2009 she travelled to the world athletics championships in Berlin with the South African athletic team to assist and treat them in their preparation for the event.

INTRODUCTION

This book aims to provide information on how to reduce injuries. It is relevant for everyone interested in staying active - from fitness enthusiasts at all levels to fitness professionals looking to improve their own performance, or the performance of the people they train. It is certainly clear that injury is no respecter of fashion and although new and exciting methods to train appear all the time within gyms the body is still subject to the limitations of its own very particular 'hardware' and 'software'. A greater understanding of both will help us to stay injury free, staying in health and fitness for longer, ideally throughout our entire movement lifespan.

DISRUPTING THE INJURY CYCLE

Most exercisers do not consider injury until it happens; those who consciously perform activities to prevent injury are in the minority. Benjamin Franklin famously said, "In this world nothing can be said to be certain, except death and taxes.", but perhaps, with the prevalence of injuries, we could throw this into the mix too. Injuries are widespread and many of us think that they are inevitable. Nowhere is the "injury happens" belief more obviously reinforced than by elite sportspeople. Numerous world records have been broken while the athlete was in some way managing recurrent pain. It is fairly easy to think of sports professionals who are routinely sitting out from competition injured. As professional sport continues to become ever more professional and sports performers more effectively conditioned, it is clear there is no such thing as "too fit to get injured." Although fitness level does matter it is not the deciding factor in injury prevention, so how else can we stay injury free?

CURRENT PREDICTORS

Current research and thinking presents some common themes for factors that increase the risk of injury, including:

- Volume of work performed. Excessive increases in the amount of exercise performed while allowing limited time for recovery
- Previous injury. A history of injury is the most significant and reliable predictor of re-injury
- The risk of errors made during sports movements as a result of fatigue

UNCONTROLLED MOVEMENT - A MISSING LINK

This book identifies and seeks to address another more recently identified risk factor: uncontrolled movement. Uncontrolled movement can be defined as an inability to control movement to 'benchmark standards' when required. It results in repetitive mechanical deformation of tissue, which can eventually lead to injury.

People need to move and, based on current levels of obesity and inactivity, they need to move more, but how they move matters to injury risk. Somebody free of pain or injury and free of uncontrolled movement could be said to be in a state of good 'movement health'. This is an optimum situation whereby injury risk is reduced as movement can be well controlled. Fundamental principles can be followed to improve movement control, therefore minimising uncontrolled movement, reducing its associated risk of injury.

STRATEGIES

Movement health can be both maintained and improved both in training environments and almost anywhere throughout the day through a mixture of four easy-to-follow strategies collectively referred to as 'Movement IQ'.

- **Awareness:** Develop an awareness of the body, movement, and movement quality.

- **Control:** Once there is awareness, movement control can be developed so that movement challenges can be met when required.
- **Varied intensity:** Develop movement control that suits the nature of the challenge. Due to the varying nature of movement performed on a daily basis, numerous layers of movement control are required.
- **Variability:** Develop many ways to solve the same movement challenge. No one strategy is the best; there is not a perfect way to move. The best strategy is to possess many movement strategies.

Improving movement health through the use of these four strategies reduces the risk of those tiresome, boring and actually quite painful things called injury.

The subsequent chapters in this book consider the importance of movement control in relation to injury risk. The first of these chapters covers information borne out of a highly divisive topic: core training. This subject has hugely influenced current thinking on contemporary injury prevention strategies but now causes many to be understandably dismissive. However, put aside any such prejudice or assumption at the mention of 'core stability' until the purpose of its inclusion is made clear. Although now a ubiquitous training modality, the research that first gave this subject life has moved on and has left core stability behind. This next chapter sets out to explore how, although the core training concept spearheaded movement control strategies, current research and understanding has moved on.

Central YMCA Health and Fitness Guides

1

LOOKING FOR THE CORE?

In the world of fitness, core training and injury prevention have become entwined. There exists a host of literature reporting on the effective use of core training to reduce injury (e.g., Caraffa et al., 1996; Fitzgerald et al., 2000; McGill et al., 2003; Myer et al., 2004; Paterno et al., 2004). So, if core training works, what is it? The term core stability is not easily defined. In some sectors its very existence is doubted (Lederman, 2009), while some have seen it as a cornerstone of their discipline (e.g., Pilates).

A BRIEF HISTORY

It used to be so simple. Exercisers used to work their abs in the pursuit of aesthetics; strong was good, muscle fatigue essential, feeling was believing. Then, things changed...

The late 1990s saw a shift in terminology, understanding, and beliefs about how to train the trunk. The continued prevalence of low back pain led researchers to inquire into the relationships between this condition and the roles of the abdominals and low back muscles. Findings were interpreted and disseminated, crossing disciplines, moving beyond the clinical to the sporting, and from the peer-reviewed to the mass media. Core stability was born, grew up, and got famous.

More recently academic literature has observed the merging of the roles of personal trainers, physiotherapists, and strength and conditioning coaches; yet, within these professions, the application of and beliefs behind core training vary enormously. The continuum presented below is galactic in scale. At one end are almost imperceptible muscle contractions performed in the clinical setting contrasted with the conditioning coaches' maximal strength workouts at the other. All claim to work the core, but is this the case?

THE CONTINUUM

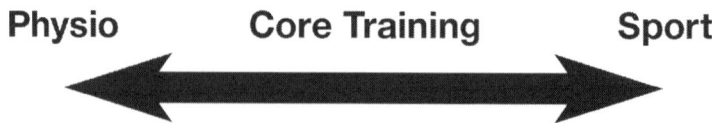

The media helps cloud the issue, tapping into superficial sentiments such as achieving an "attractive core." Sports commentators confidently discuss the top tennis player's "strong core," arbitrarily linking performance to a concept born out of therapeutic research.

Essentially, core training has an identity crisis. Some researchers (e.g., Brooks 2012) strongly question the validity of the whole approach, stating "athletes are probably wasting their valuable training time including core training in their routines." Although less damning, the Reed paper (2012) suggests that core training is effective, though only for some. These differing outcomes and opposing perspectives can be explained through an exploration of what is meant by core training at either end of the core continuum.

This search for common ground leads us to consider 'what is the core?' and what can be taken and used from these seemingly opposing worlds of rehabilitation and performance with regards to core training. Ultimately, bringing the best of both worlds together may encourage a shift in perceptions, add clarity to this controversial topic and allow for a greater understanding as to 'why' choose 'which' exercise 'when'.

WHAT IS THE CORE?

A core is the central or most important part of a thing. It is a description revealing both a locality and significance. Laptop computers have a core. Their manufacturers, eager to promote their product, set much store in the qualities of this internal hardware. However, agreement outside of technology about the definitive location of the "hardware" of the core is hard to find. For some, it will always be the internally located musculature of the lower back; for others, the term encompasses the entire trunk including the pelvic and shoulder girdles. All of these regions are in the exerciser's tools of influence – muscles. Muscles produce, slow down, and limit unwanted movement (both gross and subtle). Training can develop these qualities through the manipulation of strength (high force/structural focus), endurance (sustained, fatiguing effort focus), and skill-related (coordination) variables.

CORE COMPONENTS: "THE HARDWARE"

Certain trunk muscles have been highlighted as playing certain roles more effectively than others based on their anatomical and physiological properties. As exercise intensity changes, all muscles will be required to play their respective roles to differing degrees, a viewpoint that supports a core being comprised of the entire trunk's hardware (muscles), from the deepest to the visible. This allows exercise intensity to influence training outcomes, by placing bias on certain muscles, and peeling off or layering on muscular contributions until the correct strategy is found to bring about the desired effect.

Influential contributors such as McGill (2001) emphasise the importance of training the hardware, preferring a separation of core endurance from core strength outcomes when considering injury occurrence.

The following is an example of a hardware biased, strength/endurance exercise that targets the muscles that control rotation of the low back and pelvis. Aim to use a load that allows for fatigue within 12-15 reps.

Exercise 1: Single arm stability ball flye

With the head and shoulders supported by a stability ball in a bridge position and with the soles of the feet on the floor receive a dumbbell from a spotter into just one arm that is extended above the shoulder with the knuckles pointing to the ceiling. Ensure we have aligned the body in a mid-position and placed voluntarily contracted muscles such as the glutes and obliques prior to the start of the movement (see Chapter 3). Maintain alignment throughout the body as the dumbbell is allowed to lower out towards the floor at the side of the body in a flye action. Return with control. (See Volume 2, Chapter 2 for specifics of shoulder alignment). The greatest challenge will probably be felt in the pelvis, aiming to prevent a twisting, a challenge met by the gluteals and the obliques.

This would be an appropriate exercise for those that struggle to control the pelvis and low back during strength/endurance activities.

The hardware/strength approach, typically favoured by those from a strength training background, represents some of the demands of daily living in which both strength and endurance are routinely required. As the level of challenge tends to vary throughout a day and between individuals, movement must be controlled in many ways, as represented by the core training continuum. Strength and endurance are both sometimes the answer to a movement challenge, yet frequently another element is also required.

CORE COMPONENTS: "THE SOFTWARE"

The core's hardware is made "smart" by its "controller," the central nervous system (CNS); (part of the software in our analogy). In good movement health, a highly interdependent blend of passive (bones and joints) and active (muscles) hardware operates effectively under its control. Using a constant internal 'conversation', the software allows all components to talk and listen to one another; a discourse that aims to meet the varying challenges of the day. Just like the hardware, this software is also able to be upgraded through effective training. Motor control is a term for software-biased training and is typically favored by those from a rehabilitation background. One of the CNS's main functions, and one that is central to movement health, is muscle recruitment in which the nervous system must efficiently choose which muscles to employ, when, and how much each will contribute to any given task. Hodges & Richardson (1996) have shown that training the software can change the way the CNS responds, selecting some muscles preferentially to others.

Exercise 2: Foam roller heel taps

To make the distinction clear between a software and hardware biased exercise; try the following as a comparison to exercise 1. Lie supine on a foam roller so that the head is supported at one end and the pelvis is supported by the other as the soles of the feet are flat on the floor with the knees bent. Align the body in a mid-position throughout the trunk and then slowly lift the heel of one foot. If this proves straightforward lift the whole of the sole from the floor. Try to limit any other movement occurring apart from the leg lift. If this is an appropriate exercise it should be a manageable challenge that requires lots of attention form the exerciser. 'Hollowing' the trunk may be required to assist performance (see Chapter 3). This exercise may prove useful for those who find they have a lack of control of low back flattening at a postural/non-fatiguing intensity of work.

BODY MAPPING

The internal conversation also allows for a body to be mapped out in the brain. In good movement health each set of muscles is accurately charted, allowing for efficient movement control. In poor movement health certain regions can become over-represented, demanding excessive attention from the CNS. These high-demand regions of the body may change this map by altering the efficient navigation/negotiation of the individual's movement challenges. In such cases a software upgrade is required to redraw the map and level out the 'demanding' regions of the body.

Exercise 3: Low back (Multifidus) weight transfer

To experience an example of an exercise to change the brain map, redrawing the 'atlas' of ourselves in our head, try the following. From a standing position step forwards as if to perform a calf stretch but initially keep the rear heel down. Place the tips of both thumbs behind the body into the curve in the low back. Ensure the thumbs are as close as possible to the centre of the low back region. Now gently be.g.in to transfer bodyweight to the front foot and notice what happens below the thumbs. The muscles in this region should 'swell up' as they contract. This should happen as the movement is initiated but will be felt on one side more than the other. Now return the weight to the rear heel and feel the muscles soften. Try this again but this time concentrate on keeping the muscle contracted as the heel returns to the floor following the weight shift. The thumbs are helping the CNS find the muscle, allowing this muscle to be more represented in the brain and therefore more readily contracted. This type of exercise has been seen to assist in the rehabilitation process following back pain.

BRINGING IT ALL TOGETHER

Rather than performing just the one type of training uniting hardware - and software - biased approaches allows for a gently graded spectrum to appear; a merging of the poles of the core training continuum, from the rehab to the sporting, from the motor control to the strength/endurance. What common theme will allow such a blending?

KEEP THE CONCEPTS, LOSE THE TERM

Helping establish the link between practitioners along the core training continuum is a universal desire to control movement. An employment of the hardware under the software's control to limit, slow down or produce movement. If every use of "core stability training" was replaced with movement control the hardware or software bias debate may be defused and finally left behind. Core stability training is still packed with opposing perceptions and opinions almost religious in nature. The "what is the core" debate may never arrive at an answer. As for stability, the term is often misinterpreted; applied by some to refer to static exercises, the stability of moving systems is ignored. It is also a term that is frequently misused; exercise does not make the core more stable, it makes it more robust to movement challenges, systems are either stable or unstable, as opposed to less or more (Reeves et al., 2007).

CONTROLLING MOVEMENT, CONTROLLING INJURY

Movement control, while less catchy, is more inclusive; it spans the continuum between the clinical and the athletic. It is also highly current. Recent research has revealed how the quality of movement control in the trunk also relates to injury in the legs. In this way movement control now relates to all body regions, removing the need to mention either just the core (too confused) or just stability (too confusing).

Exercising within the movement control continuum requires choosing the correct exercise for the given movement fault. If the software is the issue we need a software solution, if the hardware needs addressing only a hardware fix will do. Without this level of specificity it is no surprise some find core training works whilst others find it just a waste of time. That movement faults can now be addressed with such specificity suggests the core debate may have proved worth having after all, if only to show how far we have come.

SUMMARY

Core training has delivered much that has taken injury prevention forwards. Some schools of thought have pursued a strength and endurance approach whilst others have developed more subtle motor control exercise protocols. Uniting all contributions under the banner of movement control allows this training approach to move forwards with greater specificity. Where once injury prevention for the trunk was the extent of this topic's influence the concept can now be expanded out to cover the whole body, at all levels of exercise intensity.

The next chapter considers the nature of the movement control challenges faced on a daily basis and how focusing on 'movement IQ' training manages them.

2

MOVEMENT CONTROL: THE CHALLENGES

The movement control continuum introduced in chapter two - connecting software (central nervous system) and hardware (muscular) focused training approaches - is now explored in more depth through consideration of the exercises identified as meeting these challenges for the trunk. Here we compare exercise intensity, the nature of movement, and inclusion of differing strategies of conscious involvement from both a rehabilitation and performance background. Some techniques may be so subtle as to be in the world of research and clinicians alone; translation movement control is one such topic. The second section deals with global movement control, a topic covering the training more commonly performed in fitness environments.

TRANSLATION MOVEMENT CONTROL

Joints are the body's hinges, opening and closing. This muscle-controlled flexion and extension of a joint is called 'physiological movement' as is rotation (twist), abduction (take limb out to side of body), and so on. This type of movement is plainly obvious, yet all is not as it seems. Although superficially opening and closing the elbow may appear to be a simple movement, where the upper arm meets the forearm the surfaces actually slide, glide and roll past each other. These are accessory movements or translation and they occur throughout the body. When a joint has none of its ligaments taut it is in a "loose pack" position, often the mid or neutral position for that joint. At this position it will move, "slop" or "translate" until the ligaments or joint capsule becomes tightened, limiting that movement.

Critical for translation movement health certain muscles play a fine-tuning, or local stability, role. In this role these structures are not producing physiological movement (flexion, extension, rotation, etc.) but are providing protection to the joint by setting a basic control of the slide and glide of translation. This may be a skill that was lost due to injury or perhaps never developed in the first place. Uncontrolled translation is related to injury due to the loss of protection that these muscles provide to the structures of the joint.

TRANSVERSUS ABDOMINIS

Under the heading of local stability muscles, transversus abdominis (TrA) is the famous muscle that made core training confusing. Researchers in the 1990s found that this muscle activated one-fiftieth of a second late in patients with back pain (Hodges & Richardson, 1996). In good movement health local stability muscles can activate prior to the performance of any movement, in any direction. Imagine a dimmer switch that turns on a light in a potentially dangerous room we are entering, allowing us to carry out our intention safely. In altered movement health we enter the room before the light turns on, which belatedly illuminates exactly what we stubbed our metaphorical toe on. Although incredibly brief, this delay is considered clinically significant and is attributable to the uncontrolled translation that occurs hundreds of times a day as any functional movements is initiated: getting up from the chair, getting out of bed, being buffeted about as we stand on our commuter train.

Following Hodges' original work hundreds of different exercises were developed to train the TrA, some of which are still in practice. Later research rendered about 70% of these exercises invalid for correcting the timing issue identified by Hodges (Tsao & Hodges, 2008). This delay is still the only reliable and consistent back pain-related change ever measured for this muscle. Clinical best practice for recovering this timing delay is just that: clinical. It is only mentioned here to demonstrate how subtle the process is and why such an approach arguably lies in the hands of clinicians.

Exercise 4: TrA bias hollowing

Recommendations for 'best practice' for recovering the TrA impairment in low back pain is to perform the non-functional low abdominal hollowing exercise to activate TrA. However do not move, or do functional activities, or loaded exercise (e.g. weight training or Pilates) at the same time. Hold the TrA exercise consistently during relaxed breathing for 2 minutes (e.g. 10 seconds × 10 repetitions) 2-3 times a day. Train in different functional static postures, with the trunk supported.

LOST IN TRANSLATION

Hodges' original work on the muscles of fine-tuning and their miniscule lapses in activation prompted many health and exercise professionals to (misguidedly) attempt to prevent back pain related to the timing delay of the TrA by using strengthening techniques. Exercises like the plank, although appropriate for challenging and improving the strength and endurance abilities of the entire abdominal wall (rectus abdominis especially), were erroneously employed for a problem related to the timing of TrA, as the strength capacity of this muscle has not been seen to be a fault related to back pain.

Also, because the timing delay is incredibly small, the need to contract the TrA during every exercise - a teaching point commonly heard in many gyms - is questioned. After the first half second or so of physiological movement, the TrA goes back to performing its role well. During a bench press, in the time required to move the hands into position on the bar the local muscles have already recruited, rendering inappropriate any cueing of this muscle during the bench press itself. No wonder there is criticism of a clinic-based technique being employed in a gym environment, and that a negative reaction to techniques originating in core training has developed across many disciplines.

GLOBAL MOVEMENT CONTROL

Following the curious world of the local muscles and the control of translation we must now delve deeper into global movement. Global movement control encompasses the movement control challenges presented by the vast majority of fitness, sport, and everyday movement scenarios. Any exercise that requires physiological movement (flexion, extension etc.) to be produced, limited, or slowed down has a global movement control bias. Through this part of the continuum exercise intensity varies from those for sustained/dynamic postural tasks all the way up to the maximal strength efforts seen in elite sport. This type of control, once enhanced, may also reduce injury.

TAKING RESPONSIBILITY - TRA OR THE OBLIQUES?

The 15 years between identifying the connection between the timing delay in TrA and back pain and qualifying how to fix it saw many back pain sufferers getting better while performing core exercises. Something must have worked. We suspect that 80% of back pain issues are related to the poor control of rotation/twisting movements. This is an issue of global control, governed by global muscles. These structures, typically more superficial than the local muscles, control bigger joints or regions of the body. Exercises that provided effective control of rotation (preventing it, producing it, or slowing it down) of the lower back and pelvis would have helped those who needed improved performance of the oblique abdominals, a key global muscle.

Many exercises that were given to back pain sufferers - and thought to be fixing the local stability fault of the TrA - were actually training the obliques. These muscles were so effectively conditioned as to actually improve back pain related to poor rotation control. The TrA sometimes took the glory for the improvements in the work of the obliques.

The next section explores how global movement control exercises meet movement challenges. Throughout, the ideas of awareness, control and variability are considered to both requisite and therefore developed.

TYPES OF MOVEMENT CHALLENGE

1. Limit movement
2. Out of neutral
3. Move through range
4. Controlling direction

1. LIMIT MOVEMENT

Some global movement exercises require movement to be limited for their duration. When performing an exercise such as the plank, the side plank, or the bridge we commonly adopt and maintain what is referred to as a neutral training region in the trunk (spine, shoulder, and pelvic girdle).

A	M - N	Z
Fully flexed	**Mid position**	**Fully extended**

Exercise 5: Finding the neutral training region

If you place your hand on the low back region and tilt the pelvis forward and backward you will notice the spine flexes (A) and extends (Z), fully one way and then the other. The middle region (M/N) is referred to as neutral. A neutral region is indicative that a place between the two end points has been found. This mid position is often suggested as an alignment less associated with injury than that of the extremes of either full flexion or extension.

It does call upon the active structures of the trunk muscles to control the body, and therefore it impacts less on the passive components (ligaments plus other structures). It is also a challenge to the software as this position must be found in multiple body regions and then maintained; possibly as muscular fatigue sets in and alters positional sense. The ability to find and hold a neutral position is a test of coordination, an indicator of the state of health of the movement system, but certainly not the end game of movement control training.

It is also important to make clear that moving out of neutral is a requirement of living. This means training needs to be performed by moving into and out of neutral, sometimes maintaining positions that are nearer to an extreme of the range.

OUT OF NEUTRAL

Exercise 6: Side plank

The side plank is a challenging exercise for many, targeting numerous muscles but often used as a means to work the obliques. Although a neutral spine may be an effective place to start the exercise we could be placing additional bias on the obliques by gently flexing the low back, posteriorly tilting the pelvis towards the "A" position. This has the additional benefit of taking effort away from the quadratus lumborum, a "barometer" muscle of movement health of the lower spine. This muscle tends to go into spasm if the joints of the low back become inflamed through injury. Excessive work of this muscle often results in an ache on one side of the lower back, associated with standing, backward bending, and habitually placing bodyweight on just the one leg.

2. PRODUCE MOVEMENT THROUGH THE RANGE

The body has many movement options: flexing, extending, rotating, bending to one side etc. All options are good if the requisite control is displayed throughout the entire range. This means moving from "A" to "Z" is necessary; performance with control is the desired outcome. For example, learning how to flex and extend the spine at different levels of intensity with excellent control is a good display of movement health/movement IQ. No one movement option is to be blacklisted or considered bad.

Exercise 7: TRX flexion-extension spinal mobility

Lie supine on floor with feet facing TRX wall mounted anchor point. Hold TRX handles shoulder width apart with palms facing one another. Using both a reverse flye like action in the arms and a curl up movement through the trunk begin to flex each segment of the spine as the body lifts slowly from the floor. Return to the floor with the reverse movement, allowing each part of the spine to touch down one by one until the start position is found again. If the aim of the exercise is simply to increase movement through any part of the spine place more emphasis on creating movement from the strength of the arms. If the trunk muscles are to be conditioned, place less emphasis on performing the movement with the arms.

CONTROLLING DIRECTION CHALLENGES

The method of movement control called direction control has been used to improve movement quality, such as with the bent knee fallout. It is performed by rotating the hip when lying on your back with the knees bent and the feet flat, so that one leg turns out while not allowing the pelvis to follow the leg.

Exercise 8: Direction control exercise

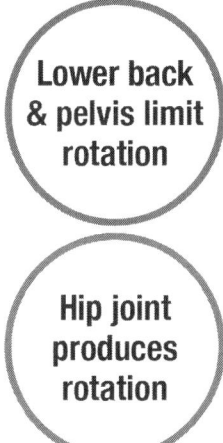

At no point is it identified that this is to be a natural pattern of movement or a functional exercise yet it has purpose. This is not a natural pattern or a functional exercise. This control sequence's progressive aim is eventually to improve function through enhanced movement quality. It seeks to improve both muscle and CNS capabilities of those muscles responsible for controlling pelvic rotation (primarily the obliques). These muscles are the masters of rotation, both its production and limitation. Control of rotation is a key component to injury prevention throughout the body, a control required in both fatiguing and non-fatiguing situations.

This exercise can be performed at various intensities depending on the exerciser's wants/needs within the movement control continuum. In this next section, intensity challenges of a non-fatiguing, postural nature are contrasted with those seen in many gym environments, from the fatiguing up toward the maximal.

THE CHALLENGE OF INTENSITY

Movement IQ requires movement control to be demonstrated at varying levels of intensity. This can be neatly split into:

1. Low intensity (non-fatiguing)
2. High intensity (fatiguing)

GLOBAL MOVEMENT CONTROL: LOW INTENSITY

Intensity matters to exercise performance and movement quality. What can be controlled at one intensity may be poorly controlled at another. The presence and nature of fatigue can distinguish exercise intensity. Additionally, where an exercise sits on this spectrum of intensity may also be differentiated through the use of conscious contractions i.e., "putting the mind into the muscle" just prior to commencing and then during the task with such methods as hollowing or bracing the trunk muscles.

HOLLOW OR BRACE?

The hollow or brace debate plagued the world of core training for a decade. The discussion hinged on whether to draw in the abdominals gently (hollow) or to contract them strongly (brace) during exercise. The answer is that it depends on what the aim of the exercise is and its intensity. Reeves et al. (2007) outline a balanced approach to the discussion, noting that situations exist during which bracing the trunk to increase its stiffness (resist movement/deformation) is critical to injury prevention (heavy, fatiguing loading in the gym) and others where a supple, loose control is required (standing/walking).

Both training strategies call upon a muscle contraction to be produced voluntarily, supplementing those occurring automatically during exercise performance. It is clear that forcing muscles to contract over sustained periods leads to fatigue and the associated pain of fatigue. Yet, there is a certain level of muscular activity, sitting at about at 5% of total effort, below which muscle contraction can be sustained indefinitely without fatigue occurring.

WORK LESS, IMPROVE MORE

We might ask what could possibly be the benefit of working at such a low intensity? If there is no fatiguing overload there is no point in the exercise, so why bother? The answer is there is an overload component in a low-intensity, non-fatiguing exercise but the overload is not physical, it is mental and biased towards improving the body's software: a "time under attention" as opposed to "time under tension strategy" (See Vol 2, Chapter 2). This approach fits the needs of movement control faults apparent in non-fatiguing situations, which also happen to make up the majority of most peoples' days. This training aims to change the brain's body map. Injury/pain may have changed this template and fatiguing exercises are not considered to improve the relevant region of the continuum at fault.

Therefore, if the aim of the exercise is related to improving posture - the ongoing battle against gravity and the demands of everyday living - the exercise needs to mimic this intensity due to the laws of specificity. Specificity states that what you do, you get better at. Those in good movement health can operate below this critical 5% threshold for many of those dynamic postural and static postural activities (standing, walking, and sitting) that must be maintained throughout the day.

Static exercises performed at this intensity can include an engaged (hollow) but loosely held mid position that avoids rigidity. Exercises that require moving regions should appear smooth, and look and feel easy. There are some good reasons for this; adopting a bracing strategy during such activities is inefficient in terms of the amount of energy spent; it doesn't make sense to employ excessive effort for something that doesn't require it. The sustained coordination tasks of posture and everyday movement are not improved through strength intensity training that requires a bracing strategy (see posture chapter). But there's more.

MAKING IT LOOK PAINFUL

Once a movement system is suffering from the effects of injury, individuals begin to use bracing strategies for dynamic and static postural intensity activities. This is evident in lower back pain patients who tend to have higher levels of inappropriate co-contraction/recruitment of trunk muscles than healthy people (Marras et al., 2001; Lariviere et al., 2002; Van Dieen et al., 2003). This has also been seen elsewhere in the body. On stepping down from a stair the gluteal muscles activate before the foot contacts the floor to assist in the control of the hip. This activity increases as the step gets higher. When contact with the floor was associated with pain, strategies normally reserved for a high step were used for the low. The body is trying to protect a region and keep it rigid to avoid pain. Deciding to copy this effect by bracing during postural-related intensity exercise teaches the CNS that this is the way to move. This would appear to teach exercisers to move as an injured person before the injury happens. Is it too far to say that this is tempting fate?

WHEN IS IT RIGHT?

Posture is a coordination task, filed under the heading of software. To change the brain (CNS) there needs to be conscious attention to the skill practiced. Attention to training quality needs to be high and muscular fatigue needs to be low in order to improve such postural-related outcomes. Simply working muscles without paying attention to the quality of performance fails to provide the appropriate training response.

GLOBAL MOVEMENT CONTROL: HIGH INTENSITY

Once muscular fatiguing effort is involved in exercise, as typically seen in the gym environment, abdominal bracing becomes appropriate due to its ability to co-contract (recruit together) more musculature. Pre-tensioning the trunk may be a desirable strategy in scenarios where perturbation force is large and expected, such as a rugby tackle or during fatiguing resistance exercises. In actuality, co-contracting many muscles simultaneously throughout the entire body becomes inevitable at such intensity. Bracing adds a voluntary element to this.

Of note, bracing is often related to breath-holding. A breath hold is perfectly acceptable for peak moments of maximum effort, say during Olympic lifting, but is definitely counter-productive when power walking on a treadmill. Yes, breath-holding does stiffen the spine, offering protection, but it is not an acceptable, efficient strategy for spinal support or movement at low intensity.

SUMMARY

Movement control is required across the full spectrum of the movement control continuum. This ranges from the subtle timing issues of the local muscles to the blatantly observable and familiar roles of the global muscles. Addressing the local stability muscles through static exercise is a task for the clinician whereas global movement control training is more suited to all movement professionals. Awareness, control, and variability can be developed with a variety of global movement exercises. It is fundamental that the intensity reflects the desired outcome of the exercise. Postural activities can be improved through exercises which focus upon time under attention, possible requiring a hollowing approach. Once strength and fatiguing endurance is required a time under tension protocol is needed, potentially accompanied by a bracing strategy.

3

POSTURE AND ALIGNMENT

It is said that "wherever you go, there you are," and so is your posture. Posture describes the relative arrangement of different body regions with a problem of a seemingly static and prolonged, yet subtly changing, movement challenge. An exerciser's posture in relation to gravity's constant influence has long been considered informative of overall movement health and this chapter considers how this is the case.

PROPORTION CONTROL

As a routine assessment, comparing the body against the fall of a plumb line can provide insight into the body's "superstructure," highlighting the distribution of muscle bulk and asymmetries suggestive of patterns of exercise, history of injury, and daily habits (e.g., whether someone is left or right handed). This subjective appraisal of the body's proportions and positioning often informs exercise selection in some movement disciplines.

For the aesthetic-focused exerciser in pursuit of a distinct symmetry, resistance training can alter proportions, adding mass to the superstructure of the body. However, if posture was simply a matter of proportion and the body only mechanically governed, resistance training could sculpt us into any shape, which we could then simply maintain throughout the day. However, both gravity and the body are a little more subtle. During the day gravity must be gently resisted, a subtle task of control for the CNS. Therefore posture is a sustained control challenge that requires the coordination of multiple body regions.

POSTURE: STATIC OR DYNAMIC

A problem becomes apparent if improved movement control is the eventual focus of a static postural assessment. From a movement control perspective this assessment may seem to capture only a snapshot of the strategy to resist gravity. Judged in this way, posture supplies only a photo, a single frame from the film that is movement.
day.

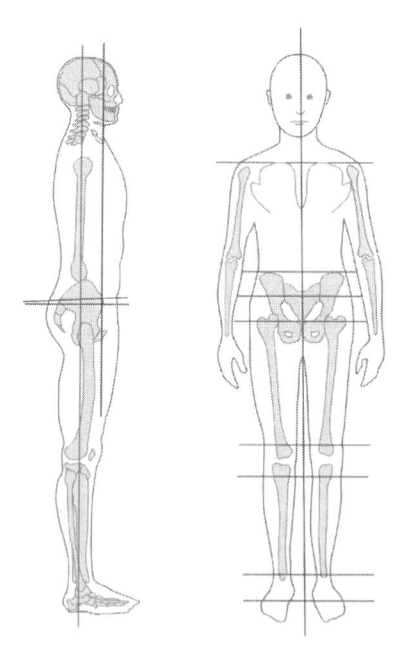

In reality posture is always in a state of flux. The body, or parts of it, are 'held' in numerous positions but only rarely is any one posture held for long. Soldberg (2005) also questions what a freeze frame postural assessment may tell us identifying numerous factors that may influence how any one individual deals with postural challenges from one minute to the next.

FACTORS

1. Emotional state - The individual's psychological factors and emotions bring about the most rapid alterations to posture.
2. Heredity - Although inherited, skeletal body type does influence postural alignment; there is also a strong link between a child's observation and subsequent adoption of the postures of their parents, even if this is not a direct blood line
3. Age and gender
4. Work environment, social factors, and physical activity

(Adapted from Soldberg, 2005)

Further clouding static postural assessment is the difficulty of removing any conscious input from the individual being tested as they think about how to stand, altering "normal" postures. All these factors combined—from the individuality of the exerciser, to their state of mind, to their understanding of the test procedure—may leave the tester questioning the value of the process.

THE TEST BECOMES THE EXERCISE

From a movement health perspective any attempt to find and hold an alignment is a display of awareness and control, two key training components of movement IQ. Static 'assessment' could be used as a training strategy to develop these qualities. However, would regularly assuming this alignment throughout the day carry any lasting benefit to movement control? What is the relationship between postures sustained throughout the day and movement health? To explore how alignment affects movement control, the concept of flexibility/range of movement must be addressed first.

FLEXIBILITY

If range of motion (ROM) is the amount of movement around the joints of the body, flexibility is the ease of lengthening of the structures through this range, allowing movement to occur. If range is the currency of movement, flexibility represents how easily this currency is spent. (See Volume 2 Chapter 3)

An exerciser's ROM in any moveable body region can be thought of as the distance between the two hands on the clock face below (A and Z).

Optimal flexibility would allow the exerciser to move from the midpoint of "12" to anywhere between "A" and "Z" with control, meeting any degree of movement challenge. Loss of active control (uncontrolled movement) anywhere in this region is believed to stress tissue and lead to injury.

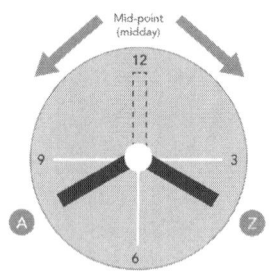

Additionally, the zone beyond "A and Z" (7, 6 and 5 on the clock) represents an excessive degree of ROM, a hyper-mobile state. Hyper-mobility has also been identified as a predictor of injury.

For some joints the mid-range (mid-day) position has been described as a desirable place from which to start training programmes for the new exerciser because it supplies a low-risk option. This region is where muscles may exert the majority of control in contrast to the "A" or "Z" position, both of which demand significant contributions from passive structures. The active structures challenged will benefit accordingly; control is required and therefore developed, and the region's passive structures (eg, ligaments) are not the primary limiters of movement. Dependent on the intensity of the activity performed this may be a loose or progressively more rigid neutral (see chapter 3).

GETTING OUT OF THE ZONE

In terms of training it soon becomes important to move our thinking beyond the neutral training region. Movement health requires movement and life cannot be lived only in a neutral position because this is not practical. Passive structures also need to be stressed through movement and its associated forces. Also, this concept would be counter to the movement variability (Chapter 1) and overarching movement health approach employed throughout this book and Volume 2.

Control is required throughout the day, both figuratively (throughout the clock face) and literally. In exercise, a mid-position is sometimes the answer. However, in day-to-day sustained postures, the ability to find and maintain mid-range positioning may be a desirable option due to how alignment influences muscle.

RANGE ALTERS FORCE PRODUCTION

Depending on where a muscle is positioned between A to Z affects its ability to produce force. In good movement health the mid-position/region (M/N) (see figure below) is the most force efficient, while at "A" or "Z" it produces relatively less force.

A B C...	M - N	Z
Fully shortened	**Mid position**	**Fully lengthened**

Postures that sustain muscles in alignments away from this mid region begin to alter the position at which the muscle is its most force-efficient. If the posture maintained is away from "M/N" and out toward "Z" for sustained periods the muscle is thought to have additional structural components added to it which causes the muscle to be more efficient at a point closer to "Z" but less effective at a position nearer to either "A" or "M/N."

A	M - N	Z
Less effective here	**Less effective here**	**More effective here**

Movement challenges between "A" and "M/N" are now poorly controlled and more prone to injury.

THE LONG AND SHORT OF IT

Cyclists provide a good example of muscle length changes that alter movement quality through habitual use. Spending many hours on a bike places the musculature across the hip region on the back of the body in a position closer to "Z." The cyclist's muscles adapt to this position, shifting their most effective force-producing point from "M/N" toward "Z." For cycling this is a good thing. However, once the cyclist needs to become a walker or runner the shift that is good for cycling becomes a movement control issue for anything in which the "M/N" or "A" position is required.

Sustained lengthening during daily postural tasks also changes where muscles produce force. The phrase "sitting is the new smoking" has relevance here for overall movement health. In terms of movement control the chair and the seated position also render these same muscles highly familiar with "Z" and unaccustomed to life and movement challenges at "A."

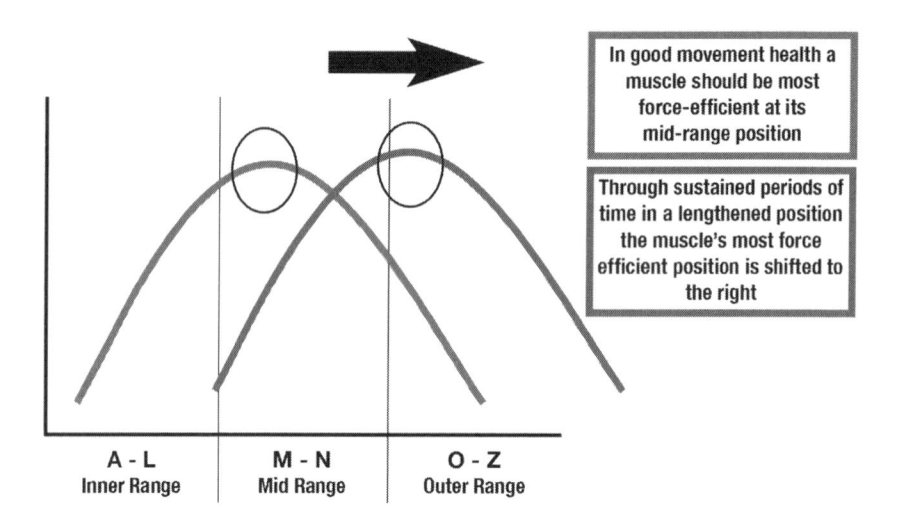

```
        →

                    ┌─────────────────────┐
                    │ In good movement health a │
                    │ muscle should be most │
                    │ force-efficient at its │
                    │ mid-range position │
                    └─────────────────────┘
                    ┌─────────────────────┐
                    │ Through sustained periods of │
                    │ time in a lengthened position │
                    │ the muscle's most force │
                    │ efficient position is shifted to │
                    │ the right │
                    └─────────────────────┘

   A - L          M - N          O - Z
 Inner Range    Mid Range     Outer Range
```

Movement control will be compromised once movement challenges are anywhere in the ROM apart from this accustomed, static point. Repositioning the body to ensure that muscles maintain optimal length and force-producing properties is one way we may alter movement quality through focus on postural alignment.

ALIGNMENT AND MOVEMENT IQ

The ability to find and hold any desired alignment requires coordination and a low but sustained level of endurance against the persistence of gravity; movement IQ demands a "will over habit until will becomes habit" approach, yet we never want to lose the ability to choose where and how we position ourselves.

The specificity of training for the sustained postural demands of the day requires time under attention challenges in the absence of fatigue. We must manage multiple coordination challenges and this is a role biased toward the CNS end of the movement control continuum.

Exercise 9: Direction control for the back

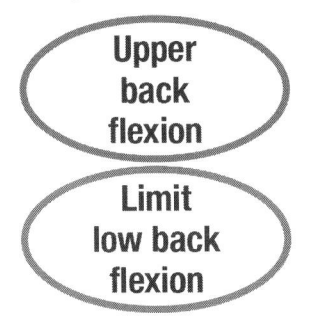

Upper back flexion

Limit low back flexion

A time under attention task to influence seated posture uses the direction control method.

From sitting, tilt the hips from "A" to "Z" and find a loose mid position (M/N). One hand can be placed in the low back curve to monitor while the other hand's first and second fingers are pointing into the body on the chest bone.

Slowly flex the upper back so that the first finger moves forward of the second, while maintaining the mid position in the pelvis and the low back curve.

Try this initially with a mirror to the side of the body but soon remove this prompt. The neck alignment is also key. Ensure any movement is only coming from the ribcage part of the spine.

Through this process we improve control at a postural level of intensity.

STAY IN THE LOOP

Another way to consider the influence of gravity is in the way it maintains muscles' activation/recruitment. Once gravity is removed muscles begin to suffer, something evident in those spending time in space. Gravity provides a sensory stimulus to the muscles that resist it, allowing the CNS to recognise these structures. The muscles respond to this stimulus by activating. If we continuously make the body map more aware of certain regions the patterns of movement and alignment associated with them become more prevalent in our everyday existence.

In good movement health the demands of gravity are shared out across the body but prolonged changes to posture can reduce the sensory prompt that is gravity to the muscle best suited to the role.

The gluteal muscles provide a good example. Routinely standing in a swayback posture (the hips forward of the rest the body) moves the pelvis sufficiently forward of the plumb line of gravity to the extent that these muscles are no longer loaded when standing.

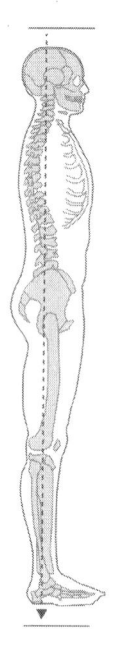

Unloading may also lead to atrophy (muscle loss) in these muscles, yet the body still needs to meet its movement challenges. The same amount of work still needs to be done yet the atrophied muscle will contribute less to the effort. In this case, the hamstrings will 'pick up the slack' making up for the less effective gluteals. These commonly overworked muscles are often described as tight and are commonly injured. Using the hamstrings in this way, in the relative absence of the glutes, often results in a clunking hip as the thigh bone is yanked backwards by muscles not best suited to the movement. Ineffective glutes will also lead the exerciser to perform lunges and squats with excessive amounts of forward lean at the hips. This increases the chances of flattening of the lower back curve, as flexion below often leads to flexion above; all of this just from standing in a very relaxed way without awareness and control.

RECRUITMENT DRIVE

Again, changing alignment can alter movement quality. Encouraging an exerciser to stand with their weight on their heels more regularly, to work on gluteal activation/recruitment, and to limit time in the swayback position may well bring the glutes back to an efficient working capacity. These muscles now need to become central to the training strategy. Anything that helps to reconnect the loop from brain to muscle is a worthy suggestion. Rothstein (1982) has forwarded the concept of a red dot reminder, a visual cue to reconnect with a more desirable alignment. Placed around the home or office, every time the red dot is seen an alignment 'self audit' is conducted. A self applied hands-on (palpation) of the desired muscle is also to be promoted. The crease between the main bulk of the glutes and the leg is the location of the region of the muscle to be targeted. The majority of time spent in a standing posture does not need a fatiguing rigidity to be employed, this crease should be a 'gluteal smile rather than a grin'.

GRAVITY AND BACKPACKS

In the same way Michelangelo cut away at the marble to produce the figure of David, gravity's presence on the body can also shape how we present ourselves. When you see people wearing backpacks, notice how the straps are pressing against the front of the wearers' shoulders and how they are responding to this. Frequently, the shoulders are pressing forwards against this area of increased pressure. The body feels the stimulus of the load and the muscles react. The muscles holding the bag demand more attention from the brain. Once the backpack comes off, the shoulders may stay pressed forward due to changes in the muscles or in the CNS, or both. We see that enhanced gravity has re-sculpted their posture. Movement control issues related to the shoulder now become apparent as the shoulder region wants to adopt this now familiar position. Finishing an upper body workout in the gym and then applying a heavy backpack to the already highly activated and swollen shoulder region could raise the risk of shoulder injury.

HOME ERGONOMICS

If shoulders hurt more at the end of the journey home than after the workout, alarm bells should be ringing. Off-loading the shoulder is easily done. Placing a large, empty plastic bottle through one of the shoulder straps spreads the loading across the chest region. The shoulder alignment discussed in the Chapter 2 of Volume 2 can now be more easily attained and maintained on the commute home, allowing any tender structures to stay clear of injury related positions. Alternatively, purchase a bag that has its own version of movement IQ. Backpacks with wheels and telescopic handles are now available, giving post-exercise users several options (on the back, wheeled left and right handed, carried left or right handed, and carried in both hands). Off-loading the shoulder works in recreation, too. We see reduced incidence of injury in golfers who use a wheeled bag compared to those who did not.

SUMMARY

Though seemingly static, the day-to-day, minute-to-minute dynamics of postural alignment may alter movement, movement quality and injury risk. Awareness and control of alignment are key tenets of movement health. Lifestyle and training options can result in an improved ability to manage the sustained presence of gravity and its effect upon the body.

FINAL SUMMARY

Volume 1 has identified the injury risk associated with uncontrolled movement, introducing the concept of movement health as a place that is free of both current injury and these movement faults. Movement IQ has been used as a collective term for methods of training that are seen to influence movement control abilities. The development of awareness, control, and variability at a range of exercise intensities can be implemented into existing exercise protocols and the changing postures of daily life. This volume has also described a movement control continuum – a spectrum that unites the sometimes opposing worlds of rehabilitation and performance.

Taking the four principles of movement IQ and applying them to warm-ups, resistance training and the development of flexibility is covered in my follow-up book *Injury Prevention: Movement control; Volume 2 warm up, strength and flexibility*. Again, based on contemporary research, Volume 2 puts a lot of the theory into a practical setting – particularly within gym environments. Discussing topics such as the employment of the RAMP method and injury risk implications of using functional movement in the preparatory part of the workout, and offering a proposed route of assessment to help clarify the murky and controversial topic of the lack of range of movement on overall movement health.

I hope you enjoyed this book, and if you wish to apply this knowledge into a practical setting, then please move on to Volume 2.

REFERENCES

Allison, G. T., Godfrey, P. and Robinson, G. (1996) EMG signal amplitude assessment during abdominal bracing and hollowing. Journal of Electromyography & Kinesiology, 8, pp. 51-57

Andrews, J. R., Harrelson, G. L., & Wilk, K. E. (2012) Physical rehabilitation of the injured athlete. Philadelphia, PA: Elsevier

Björkstén, M. and Jonsson, B. (1977) Endurance limit of force in long-term intermittent static contractions. Scandinavian Journal of Work Environment and Health, 3, pp.23-27

Blandford, L. and Comerford, M. J. (2013). What you don't know can hurt you (and your clients). Register of Exercise Professionals Journal, May. http://content.yudu.com/A1qkok/REPs/resources/index.htm?referrerUrl

Blandford, L. (2013) Movement screening: Film or a photo? Ultra-FIT, Feb/March, pp. 88-89

Borotikar, B. S., Newcomer, R., Koppes, R. and McLean, S. G. (2008). Combined effects of fatigue and decision making on female lower limb landing postures: Central and peripheral contributions to ACL injury risk. Clinical Biomechanics, 23, pp. 81-92

Briggs, A. M., Greig, A. M., Wark, J. D., Fazzalari, N. L., Bennell, K. L. (2004) A review of anatomical and mechanical factors affecting vertebral body integrity. International Journal of Medical Sciences, 1(3), pp. 170-180

Brooks, C. M. (2012) On rethinking core stability exercise programs. Australasian Musculoskeletal Medicine, June, pp. 9-14

Brughelli, M. & Cronin, J. (2007) Altering the length-tension relationship with eccentric exercise. Sports Medicine, 37, pp. 807-826

Bullock, S. H., Jones, B. H., Gilchrist, J., and Marshall, S. W. (2010). Prevention of physical training-related injuries recommendations for the military and other active populations based on expedited systematic review. American Journal of Preventive Medicine, 38, pp. 212-213

Cameron, M., Adams, R., & Maher, C. (2003) Motor control and strength as predictors of hamstring injury in elite players of Australian football. Physical Therapy in Sport, 4, pp. 159-166

Caraffa, A., Cerulli, G., Projetti, M., Aisa, G. and Rizzu, A. (1996) Prevention of anterior cruciate ligament injuries in soccer: A prospective controlled study of proprioceptive training. Knee Surgery, Sports Traumatology, Arthroscopy, 4, pp. 19-21

Cavanagh, P. R., Licata, A. A., & Rice, A. J. (2005). Exercise and pharmacological countermeasures for bone loss during long-duration space flight. Gravitational and Space Biology, 18(2), pp. 39-58

Chief Medical Officer (2010) 2009 Annual Report of the Chief Medical Officer. London: Department of Health.

Cholewicki, J., Panjabi, M. M., Khachatryan, A. (1997) Stabilizing function of trunk flexor–extensor muscles around a neutral spine posture. Spine, 22, pp. 2207-2212

Comerford, M. J. and Mottram, S. L. (2012). Kinetic control: the management of uncontrolled movement. Churchill Livingstone: Australia

Corbin, C. B. (1984) Flexibility. Clinics in Sports Medicine, 3, pp. 101-117

Drysdale, C. L., Earl, J. E. and Hertel, J. (2004) Surface electromyographic activity of the abdominal muscles during pelvic-tilt and abdominal-hollowing exercises. Journal of Athletic Training, 39, pp. 32-36

Faries, M. D. and Greenwood, M. (2007) Core training: stabilizing the confusion. Strength and Conditioning Journal, 29, pp. 10-25

Fitzgerald, G. K., Axe, M. J. and Snyder-Mackler, L. (2000) The efficacy of perturbation training in non-operative anterior cruciate ligament rehabilitation programs for physically active individuals. Physical Therapy, 80, pp. 128-140

Fuller, C. and Drawer, S. (2004). The application of risk management in sport. Sports Medicine, 34, pp. 349-356

Gabbett, T. J. (2004) Reductions in pre-season training loads reduce training injury rates in rugby league players. British Journal of Sports Medicine, 38, pp. 743-749

Gosheger, G., Liem, D., Ludwig, K., Greshake, O., & Winkelmann, W. (2003) Injuries and overuse syndromes in golf. American Journal of Sports Medicine, 31(3), pp. 438-443

Granata, K. P., Slota, G. P. and Wilson, S. E. (2004) Influence of fatigue in neuromuscular control of spinal stability. Human Factors, 46, pp. 81-91

Griffin, L. Y., Albohm, M. J., Arendt, E. A. et al. (2006) Understanding and preventing noncontact anterior cruciate ligament injuries: a review of the Hunt Valley II meeting, January 2005. American Journal of Sports Medicine, 34(9), pp. 1512-1532

Hodges, P. W. and Moseley, G. L. (2003) Pain and motor control of the lumbopelvic region: effect and possible mechanisms Journal of Electromyography and Kinesiology, 13, pp. 361-370

Hodges, P. W. and Richardson, C. A. (1996) Inefficient muscular stabilisation of the lumbar spine associated with low back pain: a motor control evaluation of transversus abdominis. Spine, 21, pp. 2640-2650

Hodges, P., Simms, K. and Tsao, H. (2009) Gain of postural responses is increased in anticipation of pain. In: Proceedings Australian Physiotherapy Association National Congress Week.

James, P. T., Rigby, N. and Leach, R. (2004) The obesity epidemic, metabolic syndrome and future prevention strategies. European Journal of Cardiovascular Disease Prevention & Rehabilitation, 11, pp. 3-8

Jonsson, B. (1978) Quantitative electromyographic evaluation of muscular load during work. Scandinavian Journal of Rehabilitation Medicine [Suppl], 6, pp. 69-74

Jull, G., Richardson, C., Toppenberg, R., Comerford, M. and Bui, B. (1993)

Towards a measurement of active muscle control for lumbar stabilisation. Australian Journal of Physiotherapy, 39(3), pp. 187-193

Karni, A., Meyer, G., Jezzard, P. et al. (1995) Functional MRI evidence for adult motor cortex plasticity during motor skill learning. Nature, 377(6545), pp. 155-158

Kavcic, N., Grenier, S. and McGill, S. M. (2004) Determining the stabilizing role of individual torso muscles during rehabilitation exercises. Spine, 29, pp. 1254-1265

Kendall, H. O., Kendall, F. P., & Boynton, D. A. (1970) Posture and pain. Huntington, NY: Robert E. Krieger Publishing

Kibler, W. B., Press, J. and Sciascia, A (2006) The role of core stability in athletic function. Sports Medicine, 36(3), pp. 189-198

Kinetic Control (2012) The Truth About Transversus: Clinical Application of the Research. Available: www.movementperformancesolutions.com/catalogue.php

Lariviere, C., Arsenault, A. B., Gravel, D., Gagnon, D. and Loisel, P. (2002) Evaluation of measurement strategies to increase the reliability of EMG indices to assess back muscle fatigue and recovery. Journal of Electromyography and Kinesiology, 12, pp. 135-146

Lederman, E. (2010) The myth of core stability. Journal of Bodywork & Movement Therapies, 14, pp. 84-98

Marras, W. S., Jorgensen, M. J., Granata, K. P. and Wiand, B. (2001) Female and male trunk geometry: size and prediction of the spine loading trunk muscles derived from MRI. Clinical Biomechanics, 16, pp. 38-46

Masani, K., Sayenko, D. G., & Vette, A. H. (2013) What triggers the continuous muscle activity during upright standing? Gait & Posture 37, pp. 72-77

McGill, S. M. (2001) Low back stability: From formal description to issues for performance and rehabilitation. Exercise Sport Science Review, 29, pp. 26-31

McGill, S. M., Grenier, S., Kavcic, N. and Cholewicki, J. (2003) Coordination of muscle activity to assure stability of the lumbar spine.

Journal of Electromyography and Kinesiology, 13, pp. 353-359

Morgan, D. L. (1990) New insights into the behavior of muscle during active lengthening. Biophysiology Journal, 57, pp. 209-221

Mueller, M. J., & Maluf, K. S (2002) Tissue adaptation to physical stress: a proposed 'physical stress theory' to guide physical therapist practice, education, and research. Physical Therapy, 82, pp. 383-403

Myer, G. D., Ford, K. R. and Hewett. T. E. (2004) Methodological approaches and rationale for training to prevent anterior cruciate ligament injuries in female athletes. Scandinavian Journal of Medicine and Science in Sports, 14, pp. 275-285

Nadler, S. F., Weingand, K., & Kruse, R. J. (2004) The physiologic basis and clinical applications of cryotherapy and thermotherapy for the pain practitioner. Pain Physician, 7, pp. 395-399

O'Sullivan, P. B., Grahamslaw, K. M., Kendell, M., Lapenskie, S. C., Möller, N. E., & Richards, K. V. (2002) The effect of different standing and sitting postures on trunk muscle activity in a pain-free population. Spine, 27, pp. 1238-1244

Panjabi, M. M. (1992) The stabilizing system of the spine. Part I. Function, dysfunction, adaptation, and enhancement. Journal of Spinal Disorders, 5(4), pp. 383-389

Parkkari, J., Kannus, P., Natri, A. et al. (2004) Active living and injury risk. International Journal of Sports Medicine, 25:209-216.

Paterno, M. V., Myer, G. D., Ford, K. R. and Hewett. T. E. (2004) Neuromuscular training improves single-limb stability in young female athletes. Journal of Orthopedic and Sports Physiotherapy, 34, pp. 305-316

Plautz, E. J., Milliken, G. W. and Nudo, R. J. (2000) Effects of repetitive motor training on movement representations in adult squirrel monkeys: role of use versus learning. Neurobiology of Learning and Memory, 74(1), pp. 27-55

Reed, C. A., Ford, K. R., Myer, G. D. and Hewett, T. E. (2012) The effects of isolated and integrated 'core stability' training on athletic performance measures: a systematic review. Sports Medicine, 42, pp. 697-706

Reeves, N. P. and Cholewicki, J. (2003) Modeling the human lumbar spine for assessing spinal loads, stability, and risk of injury. Critical Reviews in Biomedical Engineering, 31, pp. 73-139

Reeves, N. P., Narendrac, K. S. and Cholewickia, J. (2007) Spine stability: the six blind men and the elephant. Clinical Biomechanics, 22, pp. 266-274

Register of Exercise Professionals (2011) Code of Ethical Conduct. Available: www.exerciseregister.org/members/code-of-ethical-conduct

Remple, M. S., Bruneau, R. M., VandenBerg, P. M., Goertzen, C. and Kleim, J. A. (2001) Sensitivity of cortical movement representations to motor experience. Evidence that skill learning but not strength training induces cortical reorganization. Behavioral Brain Research, 123(2), pp. 133-141

Riddle, D. L. (1992) Measurement of accessory motion: critical issues and related concepts. Physical Therapy, 72, pp. 865-874

Rothstein, J. M. (1982) Muscle biology. Clinical Considerations. Physical Therapy, 62(12), pp. 1823-1830

Roussel, N. A., Nijs, J., Mottram, S. et al. (2008) Altered lumbopelvic movement control but not generalised joint hypermobility is associated with increased injury in dancers. A prospective study. Manual Therapy. Available: www.manualtherapyjournal.com/article/S1356-689X(08)00197-5/abstract

Sahrmann, S. A. (1988) Adult posturing. In: Kraus, S. I. (ed.) Clinics in physical therapy. New York: Churchill Livingstone

Sahrmann, S. (2002) Diagnosis and Treatment of Movement Impairment Syndromes. St Louis, MO: Mosby

Saner, J., Kool, J., de Bie, R. A., Sieben, J. M. and Luomajoki, H. (2011) Movement control exercise versus general exercise to reduce disability in patients with low back pain and movement control impairment. A randomised controlled trial. BMC Musculoskeletal Disorders, 12, p. 207

Soldberg, G. (2005) Postural disorders and musculoskeletal dysfunction, diagnosis, prevention and treatment. New York: Churchill Livingstone

Solomonow, M., Baratta, R. V., Banks, A., Freudenberger, C. and Zhou, B.

H. (2003). Flexion relaxation response to static lumbar flexion in males and females. Clinical Biomechanics, 18, pp. 273-279

Stokes, I., Gardner-Morse, M., Henry, S. and Badger, G. (2000) Decrease in trunk muscular response to perturbation with preactivation of lumbar spinal musculature. Spine, 25, pp. 1957-1964

STOTT Pilates (2013). 'Our Method'. www.merrithew.com/stott-pilates/method

Thacker, S. B., Gilchrist, J., Stroup, D. F. and Kimsey, C. D. (2002) The prevention of shin splints in sports: a systematic review of literature. Medicine and Science in Sports and Exercise, 34(1), pp. 32-40

Thacker, S. B., Stroup, D. F., Branche, C. M. et al. (1999) The prevention of ankle sprains in sports. A systematic review of the literature. American Journal of Sports Medicine, 27(6), pp. 753-760

Thacker, S. B., Stroup, D. F., Branche, C. M. et al. (2003) Prevention of knee injuries in sports. A systematic review of the literature. Journal of Sports Medicine Physical Fitness, 43, pp. 165-179

Tsao, H., Galea, M. P. and Hodges, P. W. (2008) Reorganization of the motor cortex is associated with postural control deficits in recurrent low back pain. Brain, 131, pp. 2161-2171

Tsao, H. and Hodges, P. W. (2007) Immediate changes in feedforward postural adjustments following voluntary motor training. Experimental Brain Research, 181(4), pp. 537-546

Tsao, H. and Hodges, P. W. (2008) Persistence of improvements in postural strategies following motor control training in people with recurrent low back pain. Journal of Electromyography and Kinesiology, 18, pp. 559-556

Van Dieën, J. H., Visser, B. and Hermans, V. (2003). "The contribution of task-related biomechanical constraints to the development of work-related myalgia." In: Johansen, H., Windhorst, U., Djupsjöbacka, M., Passatore, M. (Eds). Chronic work-related myalgia: neuromuscular mechanisms behind work-related chronic muscle pain syndromes. Sweden: Gävle University Press, pp. 83-93

Verhagen, E. A., van Mechelen, W. and de Vente, W. (2000) The effect of preventive measures on the incidence of ankle sprains. Clinical Journal of

Sports Medicine, 10(4), pp. 291-296

Wand, B. M., Parkitny, L., O'Connell, N. E. et al. (2011) Cortical changes in chronic low back pain: Current state of the art and implications for clinical practice. Manual Therapy, 16, pp. 15-20

White, A. A. and Panjabi, M. (1978) Clinical Biomechanics of the Spine. Philadelphia, PA: J.B. Lippincott

Willardson, J. M. (2007) Core stability training: applications to sports conditioning programs. Journal of Strength Conditioning Research, 21, pp. 979-985

Worsley, P., Warner, M., Mottram, S. et al. (2013). Motor control retraining exercises for shoulder impingement: effects on function, muscle activation, and biomechanics in young adults. Journal of Shoulder and Elbow Surgery, 22, pp. 11-9

Yeung, E. W. and Yeung, S. S. (2001) Asystematic review of interventions to prevent lower limb soft tissue running injuries. British Journal of Sports Medicine, 35(6), pp. 383-389

Zazulak, B. T., Ponce, P. L., Straub, S. J. et al. (2005) Gender comparison of hip muscle activity during single-leg landing. Journal of Orthopaedic and Sports Physiotherapy, 35(5), pp. 292-299

Zazulak, B. T., Hewett, T. E., Reeves, N. P., Goldberg, B. and Cholewicki, J. (2007) Deficits in neuromuscular control of the trunk predict knee injury risk: a prospective biomechanical-epidemiologic study. American Journal of Sports Medicine, 35, pp. 1123-1130

THE CENTRAL YMCA GUIDES SERIES

Happy and Healthy: A collection of trustworthy advice on health, fitness and wellbeing topics

UK
http://www.centralymcaguides.com/hhct2

US
http://www.centralymcaguides.com/hhct

The Scientific Approach to Exercise for Fat Loss: How to get in shape and shed unwanted fat by using healthy and scientifically proven techniques

UK
http://www.centralymcaguides.com/sael2

US
http://www.centralymcaguides.com/sael

The Need to Know Guide to Nutrition for Exercise: How your food and drink can help you to achieve your workout goals

UK
http://www.centralymcaguides.com/ngne2

US
http://www.centralymcaguides.com/ngne

Central YMCA Health and Fitness Guides

The Need to Know Guide to Nutrition and Healthy Eating: The perfect starter to eating well or how to eat the right foods, stay in shape and stick to a healthy diet

UK
http://www.centralymcaguides.com/gnhe2

UShttp://www.centralymcaguides.com/gnhe

Tri Harder - The A to Z of Triathlon for Improvers: The triathlon competitors' guide to training and improving your running, cycling and swimming times

UK
http://www.centralymcaguides.com/thtc2

UShttp://www.centralymcaguides.com/thtc

20 Full Body Training Programmes for Exercise Lovers: An essential guide to boosting your general fitness, strength, power and endurance

UKhttp://www.centralymcaguides.com/tpel2

UShttp://www.centralymcaguides.com/tpel

Run, Jump, Climb, Crawl: The essential training guide for obstacle racing enthusiasts, or how to get fit, stay safe and prepare for the toughest mud runs on the planet

UK
http://www.centralymcaguides.com/rjc2

US
http://www.centralymcaguides.com/rjc

Gardening for Health: The Need to Know Guide to the Health Benefits of Horticulture

UK
http://www.centralymcaguides.com/gfhh2

US
http://www.centralymcaguides.com/gfhh

New Baby, New You: The Need to Know Guide to Postnatal Health and Happiness - How to return to exercise and get back in shape after giving birth

UK
http://www.centralymcaguides.com/nbny2

US
http://www.centralymcaguides.com/nbny

The Need to Know Guide to Life with a Toddler and a Newborn: How to prepare for and cope with the day to day challenge of raising two young children

UK
http://www.centralymcaguides.com/ngtn2

US
http://www.centralymcaguides.com/ngtn

50 Games for Active Toddlers: Quick everyday hints and tips to keep toddlers active, healthy and occupied

UK
http://www.centralymcaguides.com/50uk

US

http://www.centralymcaguides.com/50us

Exercise and Nutrition 3 Book Bundle

UK
http://www.centralymcaguides.com/enb2

US
http://www.centralymcaguides.com/enb

Obstacle Racing Preparation 3 Book Bundle

UK
http://www.centralymcaguides.com/orpb2

US
http://www.centralymcaguides.com/orpb

Nutrition and Fat Loss 3 Book Bundle

UK
http://www.centralymcaguides.com/nflb2

US
http://www.centralymcaguides.com/nflb

Mums' Health 3 Book Bundle

UK
http://www.centralymcaguides.com/mhb2

US
http://www.centralymcaguides.com/mhb

Injury Prevention and Movement Control: How to Remain Active and Injury Free - Volume 1: Core Concepts and Posture

UK
http://centralymcaguides.com/inp2

US
http://centralymcaguides.com/inp

Injury Prevention and Movement Control: How to Remain Active and Injury Free Volume 2: Warm Up, Flexibility and Resistance Training

UK
http://centralymcaguides.com/imp2

US
http://centralymcaguides.com/imp

YMCA ed

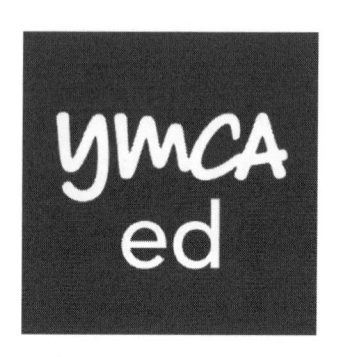

Discover more books and ebooks of interest to you and find out about the range of work we do at the forefront of health, fitness and wellbeing.

www.centralymcaguides.com

Printed in Great Britain
by Amazon